Bit
by
Bit

Bit
by
Bit

*Reclaim meaning, purpose and
pleasure in everyday life*

Colleen Rowe

Occupational Therapist

workable living
Brisbane, Australia 2017

Workable Living Pty Ltd

222/100 Bowen Tce, Fortitude Valley, Queensland 4006, Australia
Email: moveforward@workableliving.com.au

First published by Workable Living 2017

**National Library of Australia Cataloguing-in-Publication
entry:**

Rowe, Colleen, author.

Bit by Bit: reclaim meaning, purpose and pleasure in everyday
life / Colleen Rowe.

9780995436831 (paperback)
9780995436800 (ebook : kindle)
9780995436817 (ebook : epub)
9780995436824 (ebook : PDF)

1. Occupational therapy. 2. Quality of life. 3. Well-being.
4. Chronically ill--Rehabilitation

Cover design and illustrations by Natasha Smith Designs

www.workableliving.com.au

I dedicate this book to Saturday mornings:

I so look forward to our peer review group. It's a privilege to be part of an ever changing collective of people and ideas, never short of discussion about all things occupational therapy (and beyond). Your collective wisdom is a continual source of nourishment and inspiration for me.

The crossword and biting commentary of *The Saturday Paper* always provide a stimulating dose of the power of words.

And to the music-making of weekends. One of my great pleasures in life.

TABLE OF CONTENTS

Chapter 1

HOOK INTO MEANING, PURPOSE AND PLEASURE

"What day is it?", asked Winnie the Pooh.
"It's today," squeaked Piglet.
"My favourite day," said Pooh.

—*'Winnie the Pooh' by A.A. Milne*

Life's roller-coaster

Do you look forward to your everyday life? The daily grind mixed with the highs and lows; each day adding to the next as life evolves? Or have health problems or major life events stopped you from living the life you desire?

Our experiences and everyday challenges change over time, often gradually and predictably or sometimes dramatically with no warning. The speed of these changes doesn't necessarily equate to the impact they have on our lives.

A sudden injury or unforeseen change in circumstances can send you hurtling down a life-path that was not of your choosing. Equally, the slow insidious realisation of the impact of your life's challenges and choices can be bewildering and distressing. Your normal everyday life can become something you struggle to accept and enjoy.

I'm guessing that if you've picked up this book you, or someone you know, are facing a challenging time when the drudgery of everyday has overtaken the pleasures of life. Perhaps you are trying to cope with a roller-coaster of emotions, energy or pain that affects everything you do (and don't do). You may be dealing with a health diagnosis that seems to have lifted you out of the world you know, or a major life event that has blind-sided you. You may be at a point where you feel that life is, in some way, deficient, unsatisfying, and not what you had envisaged or hoped.

The good news is that to move forward in **your** life, you don't need to research the latest medical breakthroughs and treatment options. You don't need to (re)acquire new skills and you don't need to turn yourself into a pretzel trying to change the way you think about life. Instead, you can change **what you do** each day and **how you do** things to generate more meaning, purpose and pleasure in your daily life.

What is occupational therapy?

I've been an occupational therapist for 30 years, and I love that occupational therapy focuses on the doing aspect of living—on the things you *do* that *occupy* your time. Instead of concentrating on the result of your illness or circumstances, occupational therapists concentrate on the results of what you do each day.

After all, it is the outcome of your day that matters. The notion that, at the end of the day, you have a sense of achievement and satisfaction. Your day has in some way been enjoyable, fulfilling and enlightening; and you feel tomorrow has the potential to be so as well.

In this book, I'll tell you about an occupational therapy approach to living. This is based on the underlying proposition that what you actually do (or don't do) each day is the product of a host of interactions, not all of which relate to your personal skills and capabilities. These interactions are between what you do, how you do it, where and with whom, and what you want to achieve in your day. As you explore this approach, you will see that by simply changing one of these aspects, you can create a different outcome to your day.

A large part of what you'll see here explains the theory of occupational therapy. Over the years I have developed my own unique way of interpreting the theory and of using a mix of techniques and concepts with people across the spectrum of age, circumstances, and stages of life. So I'll tell you about the theory and I'll also talk you through putting that theory into practice, using terms and activities that bring the theory directly to you.

What you will discover

Our days are full of things we do, things we don't do, and all the other things we should, could or would have done. Sometimes you manage to do the things you want to do, and at other times you don't. You are more likely to do something when it is very enjoyable or when there is a very clear purpose that resonates with your expectations, hopes, and values. These are the hooks that pull you into doing the things you need to do and want to do in your daily life. In other words, it is not the tasks themselves that drive you—it's the meaning and purpose they have within your unique life. The pleasure, satisfaction and value that you derive from what you do are your hooks. Daily tasks allow you to survive, but it is the meaning, purpose and pleasure of those tasks that enable you to thrive.

This book will help you discover what hooks you into doing the things you actually get around to doing, and what is missing when you don't do things you know you "should" or "would" like to do.

Over the years, the theory and practice of all the helping professions have changed and evolved. There is no "one size fits all", yet book shelves continue to bulge with works prescribing the latest, newest, different techniques to try. The beauty of the approach in this book—my approach to occupational therapy—is that it gives you a scaffolding from which you can develop your own understanding of what is likely to work for you. By examining the context of your life's roles and activities, your expectations and aspirations, your needs and limitations, you construct your own frame of reference from which you can develop daily routines and lifestyle choices. You will find safe, healthy, efficient and inspired alternatives to make sure you are not spending all your precious energy on just surviving day-to-day.

You will also discover that you can have more control over your emotional responses to life without expending huge amounts of energy to do so. You will discover how to do things differently to lessen the drain on your emotional reserves. You will then be able to take on and sustain change without it becoming overwhelming, which will ensure you have the energy you need for the rest of your day—particularly the fun parts.

In chapters two through five I will talk you through the concepts of my approach when working with my clients. This is a crash course in the theory of occupation and a model of practice that I have adapted within my work style. I'll introduce the umbrella analogy.

In chapters six to eight I will give you a taste of what it's like to work with me in this way. I will give you some practical things to do to get you started—to dip your toe in the water of working with umbrellas.

By doing things differently or doing different things, you will have different outcomes. The approach outlined in this book will have you reclaiming meaning, purpose, and pleasure in your daily life.

Chapter 2

THE MEANING OF OCCUPATION—
AN UMBRELLA CANOPY

"If you want to build a ship, don't drum up the men to gather wood, divide the work and give orders. Instead, teach them to yearn for the vast and endless sea."

—*Antoine de Saint-Exupery*

What is occupation?

The things we do each day shape our lives and give our lives meaning and purpose (or not). What is it that makes what we do meaningful? Why doesn't putting more effort into life make it more rewarding? Will life be more satisfying if I do more or if I do less?

Occupation—from an occupational therapist's point of view—is described as the things you **do** that **occupy** your time. The theory talks about occupation as being more than just a task or an activity; it is something you do that has meaning and purpose beyond the actual activity itself. For example, the movement of picking up a pen or pencil becomes a task when you write words on a page or write a letter that communicates a message. It is only when the letter becomes a job application or a note to a friend that it becomes an occupation that has context and meaning within the broader scope of your life and has an impact beyond the here and now. More than words on a page, a note to a friend has a connection, a message, and has a very different purpose to a job application. It uses a different style of language. A note to a friend may use a colourful, decorative card instead of plain copy paper that you would use for a job application. A friendly letter will look and feel different to a job application and will elicit a very different response from the reader. Both activities require the same physical movements and language skills, but the reasons you engage in the task and the hopes of how the outcome will add to your life's experiences are vastly different. The intent and the hoped-for outcome are what turn a task or activity into an occupation.

"Doing nothing" can also be an occupation. It certainly occupies your time and, in most cases, serves a specific purpose—albeit not always achieving the result you would like. Spending long hours in bed with time passing may be exactly what your body needs in the early stages of recovery from illness or injury. It may be what your brain needs during a particularly stressful time to calm heightened emotions and to clear the fog in your head. At other times, it may be what you "do" in the hope that your brain or body will improve or change. In some cases, spending long hours in bed only serves to allow you to ruminate over all the thoughts swirling in your mind, which leaves you feeling less impressed with yourself than when you started. Similarly, standing staring out of the window at the ocean on a rainy day might be a signal of hopelessness or despair for someone who is overwhelmed with the challenges of the day ahead; whereas in different circumstances or for a different person, it may be a very deliberate form of relaxation and rejuvenation, of taking pleasure in watching the movement of nature, or becoming inspired for creative endeavours.

So we can see that it is not the task, the movement, the busy-ness or inactivity itself that creates an occupation. It is the meaning and purpose behind the activity. Simply participating in a task or activity doesn't necessarily give it meaning; it is the purpose, the context, and the hoped-for outcome that define it as an occupation. It is your occupations that give your life meaning, purpose, and pleasure.

Exploring your own occupations

The first step in reclaiming meaning and purpose in your life is to explore your own occupations—to clearly understand why you do the things you do. This isn't always obvious even on a very basic level of identifying the true meaning behind your daily routines and everyday tasks.

The meaning of an activity, at this particular point in time, is tied to what you have done in the past and why. At any point in time, you are the sum of your life's experiences, what you have done in the past, your connections with people, your values, your beliefs, and aspirations. These all come together to give what you do a particular meaning at a particular point in time. The things you do, the things you don't do, and doing nothing all occupy your time, and have different meanings in different circumstances and stages of your life.

When challenged to think about the concepts of the meaning and purpose of what you do, it is easy to skip straight to whether you are satisfied with what you've done. Has it been enjoyable, fulfilling, entertaining, and successful? This is actually the next step. You have to know why you are doing something and what you hope to achieve before you can determine if you've been successful. Only then can you decide whether you are happy with the result. This chapter helps you explore the "why" of what you do and helps you clarify some of the broad concepts of why you do things. The next chapter—the ingredients of occupation—deals with "how well".

The four categories of occupation

There are a myriad of things we do throughout our daily lives and a multitude of reasons for doing them. To simplify the process of exploring your own occupations, you can divide all the things you need to do and want to do into categories based on meaning and purpose—the theorists call these categories "occupational domains". Note the use of the term "occupational", which signifies purpose, context and intent; not task or activity.

If you've been in a hospital or rehabilitation facility in Australia you will probably be familiar with people talking about your self-care, domestic tasks, and community tasks; or self-care, productivity and leisure. These are some of the categories that occupational therapists have traditionally used and they have become part of the language used by health and support services.

However, the concepts of how we categorise occupation have changed over the last decade, partly because of the evolving nature of lifestyles and community services. It is true also that the naming of categories, such as those mentioned, has tended to draw together a set of specific tasks rather than bring together an over-arching idea of the purpose and value of activities. In naming my categories, I have, therefore, used terms that relate to intent and not to groupings of tasks or of places (home, community, work). When categorising your occupations, it is important to always keep in mind meaning and purpose, not movement or activity.

In this book, I use four domains of occupation based on four very broad categories of the reasons we do things. The four categories are:

- Survival and Health
- Connecting and Contributing
- Leisure and Learning
- Rest and Recuperation.

Survival and Health

Survival and health tasks are the things we need to do to stay alive and healthy—food, water, shelter, warmth and hygiene. The survival tasks include getting showered and dressed, preparing and eating meals (including shopping for same), organising and paying for appropriate accommodation, managing medications and other activities that help maintain a healthy physiology—not forgetting collecting the mail and dealing with the rubbish, paying bills, managing laundry and house cleaning. Conceptually all these tasks relate to health maintenance—if you don't do them on a regular basis, be that daily, weekly, or annually, then you will eventually become ill.

The literature variously calls this self-care, health maintenance, self-maintenance, self-help—all of which have been bandied around by different professionals in different contexts and which no longer have a clearly defined meaning. In particular, the term "self-care" is used by so many different people and organisations in vastly differing contexts that it is often difficult to know exactly what is meant. So I prefer to use the term survival and health to signify the tasks' purpose.

These tasks are often centred around the home, but not always. Particularly over the last decade as the internet has changed our lifestyles so significantly, daily tasks that were previously "home-based" or "community-based" have shifted their geographical base for many people and for changing lifestyles. This is another important reason to understand the domains and not restrict your thinking to traditional geographically-based activities or standard lists of tasks. The survival and health tasks are the things you need to do to stay healthy, regardless of whether you want to do them or not. They are the tasks that create a healthy physiology that, in turn, forms the basis on which you can engage in the other three categories.

Connecting and Contributing

This category is the things we do that contribute to society and connect us to our community. While the first domain, survival and health, relates to our own health and survival, this category relates principally to other people. It describes our connections with other people and our place within society; contributing, participating, connecting with others, creating families and communities, fostering cultural continuity.

This is the category where most people would include paid work; although some might be tempted to put work in the survival domain if they view their work as purely a means of funding the rest of their life. Remember that in categorising the things you do, you look at the intent of your involvement in the task, not your satisfaction or enjoyment—looking at those aspects comes later. Work connects us to a community. Even if you work from home sitting alone at a desk, you still connect in some way to people through work and work contributes to society. Commercial interactions of any nature have an impact on other people. Regardless of whether you enjoy your job, or whether you feel fulfilled or energised by it, it is fundamentally a connection to society.

This category also includes our family roles and relationships. These are the things we do to care for other family members, parenting and ensuring our children are safe and healthy, activities that create the bonds of families. It also includes our involvement in community groups, sporting clubs, cultural activities, and gatherings of friends. These are the things you do to express your aspirations in life and that reflect your values. In previous literature, this was often referred to as "work" or "productivity"; but again these words mean different things to different people, particularly in the political and commercial world. This category exemplifies the richness of experience, pleasure and reward from interactions with others, an outcome that has value to others and activities that foster relationships and communities.

Leisure and Learning

The third domain is leisure and learning. These are the things that provide pleasure and inspiration from the activity itself rather than from interactions with other people. These tasks are opportunities to engage your creativity, to learn and develop new skills, to do things purely for self-satisfaction and self-advancement. In other words, 'me-time'—even though the me-time might be spent with other people. If you enjoy landscape painting you might choose to sit in your backyard while drawing aspects of your garden or you could join a group of artists who gather in your local park. There might be very little discussion while everyone paints or there might be lively banter (art related or not). Or you might join a more formal art class and have individual tuition or group lessons. Each of these activities will fulfil your pleasure of painting and provide leisure and learning; they have varying degrees of connections and social interactions with others. But they are all 'me time'.

There's no limit to the activities that can fit into this category—what matters is what they mean to you at this point in your life.

Rest and Recuperation

Finally, the fourth domain is rest and recuperation. This domain recognises the need for good sleep patterns and the importance of sleep to manage all the other areas of our daily life. It's very difficult to function well throughout the day after a poor night's sleep, particularly after a succession of nights of poor or interrupted sleep. Tied in with sleep is your ability to relax and to recuperate, to have a break from the other three categories, to re-energise or to be calm. This is a category that is often missed by health professionals and is generally not well "treated" within our current health systems, and yet it has an enormous impact on all other aspects of our lives. This category looks at your sleep habits and patterns, whether you wake feeling refreshed in the morning. It looks at your ability to recognise your need for rest, and what you do to recuperate (physically as well as emotionally) and re-energise. It is the category that incorporates the things you do and don't do to soothe and be calm.

Same task—different domains

A particular task could fall into different domains for different people or fall into more than one domain for the same person. Cooking is a good example of this. Food preparation is part of the survival domain—we need to eat to stay alive; we need to have a healthy diet to maintain optimal health. Even if this simply involves going to a café or buying pre-prepared meals, there is still time and effort needed to do this. For some people, cooking is simply something that has to be done each day; for others it is a pleasure, part of the me-time, a time to relax, to be by yourself, to think and ponder (or not), to be stimulated by all the colours and smells and textures of food. For others, it is an integral part of family life and family connections—part of the role of providing for other people's needs, or a regular opportunity to talk about your daily happenings with the people you care most about. It may be your creative bent, an opportunity to experiment, to learn (or teach). It may be your profession or your livelihood that is a means to a different end. And so the same activity has a different meaning and purpose for different people and may be in more than one category, or may be in different categories at different stages of life.

So we see that it is not the activity or task or role *per se* that helps categorise the things you do, but the meaning those things have to you individually within the context of your daily life and lifestyle at this point in time. It is the purpose that a particular task or activity serves in the overall picture of your life.

Your umbrella canopy

When you collate all the things you do that occupy your time, and separate them into the four different domains, they collectively form an overarching picture of your life's meaning and purpose.

They create an umbrella of the meaning of the things you do that occupy your time.

A crucial feature of any umbrella is to have a complete canopy over your head. Just as an umbrella with only one section of fabric is little use on a rainy day, the umbrella of meaning and purpose is only useful when it covers all four domains. When you know that you are not spending all your energy on just surviving day-to-day; when you recognise the importance of connecting with people around you and with your community, of having time and resources for leisure and learning and opportunities to recuperate and re-energise.

When you are consciously aware that survival tasks might not be enjoyable but are maintaining your health, they become more doable. Especially when you can clearly see other activities in your umbrella that provide you with pleasure and satisfaction. Having a clearer understanding of why you do things, and which activities provide enjoyment and vitality can help you prioritise where to spend your time and energy. This will hook you into doing more of the things that give meaning, purpose and pleasure to your every day.

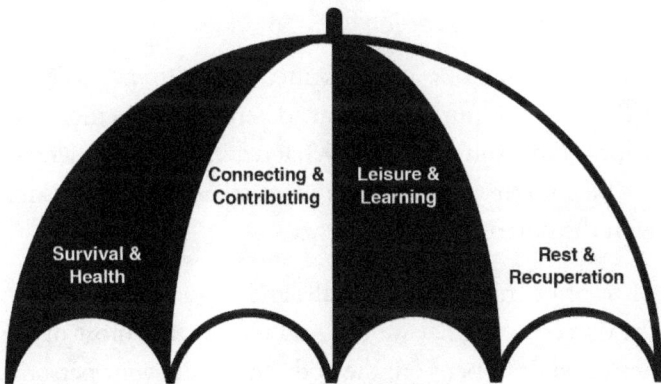

Connecting & Contributing

Leisure & Learning

Survival & Health

Rest & Recuperation

Chapter 3

THE INGREDIENTS OF OCCUPATION— THE UMBRELLA SPOKES

"I can't change the direction of the wind, but I can adjust my sails to always reach my destination."

—Jimmie Dean

What are the ingredients?

When you set out to do something with a particular meaning and purpose, what determines whether you achieve the result you want? What determines whether you get pleasure from doing it, and whether you are satisfied with the outcome?

Most of us think that our skills and capabilities influence the outcome of what we do. And this is what most of the health services focus on; the body and brain, your personal abilities. However, the things you do, where you do them, and how you do them don't operate in isolation. The difference with an occupational therapy approach is that we not only look at your personal skills, but also at the environments in which you do things and the characteristics of the task itself, and put these together as an interactive model. These three ingredients of your occupations interact to produce an outcome—not only the result of the activity, but whether the purpose has been achieved and if it's been enjoyable and worthwhile.

Once you have more clearly defined why you do the things you want to do and need to do (your umbrella of meaning), only then can you analyse whether you are satisfied with what you actually do. The domains help you hook into meaning and purpose. The ingredients are the factors that produce the outcome and therefore determine satisfaction and pleasure.

In other words, it is the interactions of these ingredients of occupation that determine the nature and quality of the outcome. This is not simply a "yes/no" response to interminable lists that ask, "Can you do . . . ?" Living is about so much more. The questions that should be asked are: Do you enjoy what you do? Do you feel safe? Does it matter if you do it well? Can you consistently do things when you need to, and do you have the energy and resources to do them when you want? How useful is this? Is it valuable or rewarding?

Returning to our umbrella analogy, these are the spokes that hold up the canopy. You need an integrated system of spokes to hold up your umbrella, to keep it open and provide cover from the rain. It doesn't really matter what the spokes are made of as long as they are strong enough and plentiful enough to collectively keep the canopy firmly aloft.

The interactive model

In this chapter, we'll look at the details of the ingredients—the factors that influence the outcome of what you do, and how they all interact to determine your pleasure and satisfaction. We'll look at the three types of factors that make up the PEO model of occupational therapy practice—Person, Environment and Occupation. Firstly, we'll look at the details within each category and then we'll look at how they interact to produce the result you want (or don't want).

When you are able to analyse the different ingredients of what you do (this is what occupational therapists call task analysis), you can look at changing some of the ingredients to change the outcome. Sometimes this will involve swapping some of the factors that used to work for you with different factors (different types of umbrella spokes) that can still produce a gratifying result. In other instances, it might involve looking at a completely different outcome that produces the same meaning and purpose.

This way of working helps you understand the interconnections of all the factors and then to anticipate what changes can be made to make your way of living easier and more achievable and, therefore, have a life style that is more workable and enjoyable for you. This is quintessentially occupational therapy.

Person

The first ingredient is the Person. This is your physiology; your body and brain working together. It is how you move, how you think, how you feel—your body systems and functions. It is your person that most health professionals work with and, in the acute stages of illness or injury, this is where the main focus should be—on correcting your physiology where possible and working on early recovery of skills and capabilities.

Your person acts as a system of elements that affect each other, a continuum of responses within your body and brain. Your body senses something—you hear the sound of a car approaching very fast, your stomach rumbles, you see a familiar face in the shopping centre, you smell burning toast, you feel a dull aching pain in your back, you think a fearful thought. Your body (usually your brain, but not always) receives the signal and makes sense of it— what does it mean? What needs to happen? And then your body responds with movement, thoughts or metabolic processes. This produces an outcome that triggers another set of sensory input for your body and brain to deal with. Your brain is constantly filtering and managing this round-the-clock inflow of sensory information, consciously or unconsciously and even when you are sleeping.

In the context of the things you do in your daily life, your responses are generally what we call your skills and abilities—your body sensing, analysing and then acting. Let's take the example of a car approaching fast as you walk across the road. If you have sharp hearing and clear vision, your body will send sensory messages to your brain about the car approaching (speed, estimated time of arrival) which it will start to analyse. If you have well-developed cognitive skills, your brain will instantly recognise the danger and send messages to your muscles which will enable you to quickly get out of the way of the car provided your nerves and muscles work well. The end result is that you have the ability to cross the road safely.

However, a change at any stage of the process will change the outcome, and, therefore, alter your skills and abilities.

At the sensory stage, if your hearing is impaired your brain won't receive the correct auditory information to analyse the danger and respond accordingly. But if you correct the sensory input by regularly wearing a hearing aid or using your vision as a substitute, you are able to send sensory information to your brain which will enable you to get out of danger.

At the analysing stage, if you are highly distractable your brain might not focus on the urgency of the situation; or if you have difficulty filtering through all the possibilities and scenarios you might not create a plan of action quickly enough. And so while your hearing may be perfectly fine and your legs work very well, you don't jump out of the way of the car in time.

And at the action stage, if you have a broken leg and are using crutches, your ability to take the action that your brain wants is limited and, in this instance, you are potentially very unsafe. You will be safer crossing the road if you are more vigilant in looking and listening before crossing the road, and cognitively making sure you have more time than usual. If you use the sensory input and analysing stages to compensate for your decreased output skills you will be safe crossing the road.

Your body and brain are constantly responding to the world around you—to the people and places, to your thoughts and ideas, to the outcomes of the things you do. Just as your occupations sometimes involve doing something and sometimes doing nothing, your responses are sometimes movements and actions and thoughts, and sometimes not.

Let's look a little more closely at this body-brain continuum and look at some of the factors that can change over time.

The three stages of body-brain continuum

During the first part of this body-brain continuum—the sensory input—your body receives lots of information in addition to the classic five senses (hearing, vision, taste, smell and touch), for example temperature, pain, balance, the position of your joints, hunger and thirst. All this input is constantly being analysed. Sensory input can change over time. A musician can develop very acute hearing, whereas a factory worker may have dulled hearing from constant noise. Playing sport can improve your body position sense.

Vision and hearing tend to decrease as we age. Senses can be damaged by injury or illness—a nerve injury or diabetes can alter touch and temperature sensations. Some people are over-sensitive or under-sensitive to certain sensations and the information sent to the brain is muted or intensified and, therefore, can be more difficult to interpret. Pain sensations change over time, especially with chronic pain. Any changes in any of your sensory pathways will affect whether you make sense of the information, how you plan to deal with it and what responses you will have.

The second stage—making sense of your sensations— requires a complex network of sensory processing skills, cognitive skills, emotional and social skills. This is your brain's ability to correctly interpret the information it receives, to think clearly about what is happening and come up with a viable plan. Your ability to make sense of the input from the world around you and decide what to do about it is constantly changing over your lifespan, partly through the natural processes of developing and learning, and also when illness or crisis happens.

These are cognitive skills you develop over your life span— perception, insight, attention span, memory, doing things in a timely fashion (to name just a few!). They also include the ability to communicate effectively with people, to understand what responses are appropriate for a situation, your belief in your own capabilities, your emotional regulation, how your ethics and values influence what you do.

Equally as complex are the various ways these skills can be changed, improved or impaired throughout your life. There is certainly a plethora of injuries, illnesses and life-long diagnoses that can change the physiology of your brain. Hormones and stress add different chemicals to your brain physiology and are factors we will all deal with at some stage. Your life's experiences will also have an impact on the way your brain analyses the information it receives, your emotional responses to life, memories of past events and associated after-effects.

The changed thought patterns of someone who has depression, anxiety or a phobia may impair their ability to go down the street to do the shopping despite their sensory input and muscular skills being completely intact. Someone who is very distractible and has difficulty focussing attention for long periods of time may have difficulty completing a jewellery project despite having very good dexterity and creative skills and deriving enormous pleasure from this artistry. The fear of pain can alter what we choose to do.

The third part of the process is the output. Nerves, muscles, bones and joints all working together provide coordinated movement. Healthy heart and lungs feed your muscles. Balance and dexterity, speech and thoughts all work together. Any injury that affects muscles and joints will have an obvious impact on your "output" skills. If you have chronic lung disease, your ability to walk long distances will be noticeably reduced, as will the more obvious impairment of a leg injury. A stroke or head injury may affect your ability to walk, to use your arm and hand, to talk and communicate, or to think clearly, depending on what part of the brain is affected. Your dexterity may improve as you practise piano every day; your thought patterns may become more encouraging as you practise deep breathing exercises.

The combination of input, analysis, and output produces your skills and capabilities. The complexities of body and brain work together to produce an outcome—a movement, thought, behaviour, activity, or inaction. Your body and brain constantly changes over your lifespan—the developmental stages of childhood, adult study and work, social interactions and changing family roles, illness and injury that can be temporary or long-term. These all affect one or more stages of the input-analysis-output continuum. This is the person ingredient of occupation—the first of the three categories of ingredients.

Your person and all the complexities of body and brain is what you will most likely concentrate on during the initial stages of an accident or illness. Even in the absence of illness, during the initial stages of a crisis or an unexpected life event you may concentrate on shoring up your emotional responses and clear thinking to work your way through good decision-making. But after the initial stages of a crisis, or when the acute phase of an illness or injury has finished and you are returning to home life, the other occupational factors of environment and occupation come into play.

Environment

The second ingredient of your occupations is the environment in which you do things. We live in a multitude of different environments that all interact to influence what we do and how we do it. Perhaps the most tangible is the physical environment, which is the geography of where you are—the combination of the built environment, the natural environment, places and spaces. Examples of how the physical environment influences our daily lives are: the difficulties that stairs or uneven ground impose on someone who has difficulty walking, poor vision or is pushing a stroller; the benefits of lots of natural light in the home of someone who has depression in contrast to dark, dingy rooms; a well-fenced open space providing safety for a child with an over-abundance of energy; the facility of good seating in a shopping centre to ease fatigue and facilitate conversation and connections within the community.

We also do things within emotional and social environments—the people around us, our connections and relationships with them. The pleasure you derive from cooking a family meal is influenced greatly by the reactions of the people who eat the meal—their compliments, appreciation, criticism or ambivalence may also affect how you go about cooking another meal tomorrow. You might accidentally cut yourself when preparing food while you are very emotionally upset or distracted by people around you even though your physical skills (your person skills) are perfectly capable of using a knife without incident and haven't changed since yesterday. It's difficult to get out of bed in the morning when it seems as if the drudgery of getting through the day is all that lies ahead, whereas waking with the realisation that today is the day of a much anticipated event instantly makes it easier to get up and going. These are all examples of the influence that the social and emotional environments can have on the outcome of what you do, as well as the effect they have on your satisfaction and enjoyment.

The economic, cultural, organisational, and political environments also influence what you do, how you do it, and the outcomes of your actions and activities. The music you listen to and your style of dance is likely to be influenced by your cultural connections. Having a stable income will have a big influence on your choice of home and other lifestyle options. The "rules" of your local library will guide how much noise you make while browsing the book shelves. And so at any particular time and place there are multiple environments determining and shaping the outcomes of the things you do.

Think about a time when you sat down with a book to read. There are multiple environments that affect the ease, comfort and enjoyment of your reading. The chair design and cushioning will affect your comfort; the height of the seat will influence the ease of getting in and out of the chair. Good lighting will help you see the page without shadows. The temperature surrounding you will affect your enjoyment—an air-conditioned room on a hot summer's day, a cool breeze while sitting in the park, sitting in front of an open fire while it snows outside in contrast to a cold empty room. You will be affected by neighbours using a chain saw to do their tree trimming or a quiet neighbourhood with bird song, being able to choose to listen to music or having someone else's music imposed on you. Part of the environment is your choice of book—favourite authors and engaging subject matter versus reading because you 'have to'. Reading political commentary or cartoons that are current versus historical will likely provide a different experience. Family members arguing around you, delicious smells wafting in from the kitchen as someone else cooks your dinner or the smell of burning toast may affect your enjoyment. None of these environmental factors change your ability to sit and hold a book, to read, interpret, and understand language, i.e. your person skills. They may change whether you are able to concentrate in that place at that time, but they don't change your personal concentration skills. They all change the outcome, in particular your level of enjoyment.

You can make deliberate choices about some of your reading environments to change the outcome and enhance your enjoyment (your choice of chair, being inside or outside, in the middle of the family melee or in a quiet retreat). Other parts of the environment, such as the neighbour using the chain saw, are not entirely within your control.

It's not always possible to change the environment, but there are a surprising number of ways you can alter it. If you have difficulty bending, you can place the most frequently used kitchen items and utensils within easy reach so that food preparation is less painful and strenuous. If you have difficulty walking for prolonged periods of time, you can lobby for seats to be installed in your local supermarket to ease fatigue when shopping. You can turn off distracting music or change to a different style of music while working. You can encourage appreciative comments from your family at the dinner table to increase your enjoyment of providing meals for them. Being with different people will change the social and emotional environment that surrounds you. Changing the environment will change the outcome of what you do without needing to change your person skills.

Environments are essentially the context in which you do things. The numerous environments interact to provide a layered context to the things you do. Your financial environment will affect how you manage any accessibility challenges in the physical environment of your home— whether you can afford to make changes to the layout or whether you can move to or build a more accessible home. Your family environment—how close you are to your extended family and how much your daily lives are intertwined—will affect your emotional environment of support, care, attention, and affirmation. Your work culture, particularly if you work in the public service, is influenced by changing political environments; even the physical office environment of a government agency can be changed as a result of political decisions.

Environments—the context of where you do things— will influence the outcome of the things you do, and will, therefore, help determine your level of satisfaction and enjoyment.

Occupation

The third ingredient is the characteristics of the occupation itself—the way you go about doing things and the implications of what you hope to achieve. The methods and strategies you employ to do particular tasks, how efficiently you do them, how safe your method is and how long you take to do a task will all affect the final outcome. The meaning and purpose—your intended outcome and what you hope to achieve—will influence how you perceive the outcome, and, therefore, how satisfied you will be with the result.

We all know there are different ways of doing the same task. If you are looking for a car parking space at the shopping centre, do you drive up and down the rows looking for a vacant spot? Do you scan along each row as you drive along the head row? Do you look for someone coming out of the shopping centre and follow them to their car? When you make a cup of coffee, do you use a coffee machine or use instant? Do you add milk first or last? The different car parking strategies will all (hopefully!) find you a parking spot. The way you go about making a cup of coffee will be very influenced by your personal taste preferences. Different ways of doing a task, often based on what has worked for you in the past, produces a result that you hope will match your expectations.

It is self-evident that doing things in a different way can change the outcome. But it needs to be explicitly said so that you can consciously and deliberately use this to change the outcome of activities that are challenging from other perspectives, particularly where the person factors have changed as a result of illness or injury. By exploring different ways of doing things and how this will influence the outcome, you can use occupational factors as a deliberate strategy to achieve the outcome you want.

Meal preparation is again a good example to illustrate these points. If you are preparing a meal purely as a survival task for yourself only, your cooking style and methods are likely to be very different than when you are preparing Christmas lunch for the extended family. Preparing a survival lunch may require no more preparation than opening the fridge to see what is available to put in a bread roll. Whereas preparing a Christmas feast may involve poring over cookbooks, sending emails back and forth between family members about who will bring what, and ordering specialty foods in advance. The actual "doing" of your survival lunch will be very different to how you go about producing a Christmas meal.

You might be able to very efficiently produce a cheese sandwich, but your level of satisfaction with cheese sandwiches for an everyday lunch will be very different to your satisfaction with preparing cheese sandwiches for Christmas dinner. Same task, same physical outcome, but a very different sense of achievement because of the different meaning and purpose of preparing that particular meal.

In making your cheese sandwich, there are different ways of going about this task: you might choose to buy sliced bread, sliced cheese and skip using butter; some people prefer to gather all the ingredients before starting the sandwich while others fetch things as they go; grated cheese or thick slices; salad, meat or egg as extras; bagel, crisp roll or sliced bread. These all produce different tastes and textures, and a different physical outcome. The method you choose will be influenced by the other ingredients of occupation, e.g. hand dexterity or concentration span (***person*** ingredients), your weekly food budget or your cultural influences (***environment*** ingredients). And your personal taste preferences will also play a big part.

Different ways of doing things require different physical movements and different thinking skills. So the way you go about doing a particular task can have different results, even though your own abilities haven't changed. Buying off-the-rack clothes from the local shopping centre will produce a very different result to buying fabric and sewing your own design. The method you choose will first depend on the purpose of the task—whether the main reason is to engage in a creative process or whether you simply require some clothes. It might depend on how well your sewing and creative skills match the type of outfit you want. Or it might be dictated by time constraints or budget. Each method requires very different physical skills, as well as different thinking and creative skills. They require different amounts of time and energy and will produce a very different sense of achievement and satisfaction—same task of "acquiring clothes", different purpose, context, and outcome. One is not necessarily 'better' than the other;

they represent different methods of going about a task in different circumstances and for different reasons.

As with the other ingredients, the characteristics of occupation have many aspects to them, some a lot more obvious than others. The way you go about doing things often changes as your life evolves.

Another characteristic of occupation is time. Some of the things we do are very dependent on being able to do them in a certain amount of time. Ask a 100-metre sprinter how much difference 1/100th of a second makes in an Olympic race. For a farmer in the middle of the harvest season 1 minute may not make a lot of difference, but 1 hour or 1 day may be crucial. Serving up a hot meal has time constraints in terms of being able to sit down and enjoy it before it gets cold. Other meals that are served at room temperature are not so reliant on time during the preparation and serving process. There are other tasks where taking extra time to get detail and precision correct is very important. Tai Chi exercises require slow, controlled movements to achieve maximum benefit; the slow movement of a piano sonata demands time and nuance even though you may be physically capable of playing it three times as fast.

Time is also important within the context of the whole day. A particular task or occupation may not matter if it takes a long time, but in the context of all the other things you want and need to do, taking a lot of time to do one task may influence your enjoyment of the day as a whole.

Another important aspect of looking at the characteristics of occupation is to look at different activities that achieve the same meaning for you within the context of this current stage of your life and lifestyle. We tend to do this automatically throughout life with sporting and outdoor types of pursuits without thinking "different activity, same meaning and purpose". The way we participate in sports tends to change as our bodies age even though the fundamental purpose remains the same. Our hobbies and leisure pursuits (the leisure and learning domain) evolve as we move through different life stages (principally in response to time and money available). So the activity you choose to achieve a particular meaning, purpose, or pleasure can change as your circumstances and stage of life also change.

The characteristics of occupation are not only the methods you use. Timeliness, accuracy and the occupational meaning of the activity will also influence the outcome. How well you think the outcome matches the intended meaning and purpose determines your level of enjoyment and satisfaction.

Interactions—strong umbrella spokes

These three broad categories of influencing factors interact to produce the outcome of what you do. There are interactions within each category, as well as interactions between the categories. The crucial point is that it is the combination of factors from each of the groups that produces a result—not just the way your body and brain function. Therefore, and here's the really important point, you only have to change the ingredients from one of the groups to change the result, to have a different outcome that better aligns with your intended meaning and purpose, hopes and aspirations. This immediately gives you a threefold wider scope for change than if you were to concentrate only on your person, on your physiological or psychological skills.

If you've had an injury or illness, or a long-term health diagnosis or an unwelcome change in circumstances, the initial stages are often spent dealing with the immediacy of the situation and having as great an early recovery in your person as possible. However, when you return to daily living, all of life's influencing factors come into play and the health of your body and brain aren't the only things that determine how you manage daily life.

This approach gives you a framework to look at the interactions of all the factors and helps pinpoint the factors that can most easily be changed to produce your desired outcome for your everyday life. By starting with a review of what you do that gives meaning and purpose to your life— the umbrella of occupation—and looking at how all of the ingredients shape the degree of fulfilment and enjoyment you derive from the things you do—the umbrella spokes— you can make small changes that aren't overwhelming and don't take all your energy. This is fundamentally what sets apart the occupational therapy approach to change; you can open up a whole range of new possibilities by looking at all the influencing factors of person, environment, and occupation. And take the pressure off your body and mind.

To move forward, you only need to change one aspect of your person, environment or task.

Looking down on the top of an umbrella you don't always see the spokes, but you know they are there when the umbrella canopy is open. You don't necessarily know what the spokes are made of or how many there are; what matters is that the canopy stays open. This book is designed to help you understand the most important and meaningful aspects in your daily life (as distinct from what you actually currently do) and then to help strengthen the spokes (the ingredients) to ensure your umbrella can stay open. Maybe you'll find ways to replace some of the "person" spokes with environment or occupation spokes.

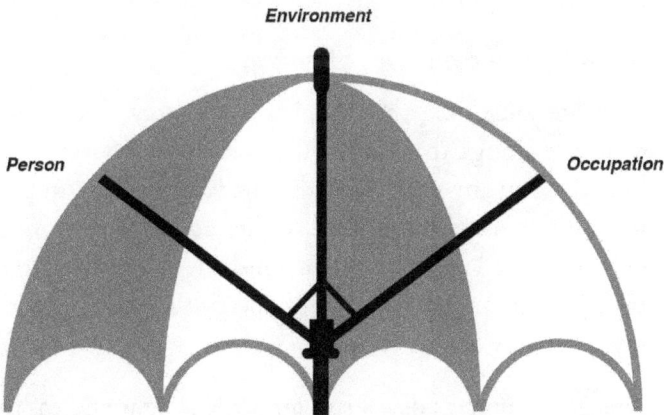

Chapter 4

ENERGY—HOLDING FIRM TO THE UMBRELLA HANDLE

*"It's no use to go back to yesterday because
I was a different person then."*

—*'Alice's Adventures in Wonderland' by Lewis Carroll*

Exploring the dynamics of energy

There are some tasks that simply drain energy. They tend to be the things that are in the survival category; they don't give you any particular pleasure; you do them simply because they need to be done. Other activities leave you more energised when you are finished than when you started. Some tasks take a lot of energy to get going and others are very easy to start.

On a still summer's day, a sun umbrella is light and easily handled as you hold it at different angles throughout the day while the sun tracks across the sky. But in really wild weather, it takes a lot of effort to hold on to your umbrella; a sudden gust of wind can pull you up short and have you trying to make adjustments before the umbrella blows inside out. In driving rain, it's sometimes hard to figure out which direction to point your umbrella. Different types of weather require different amounts of energy to hold your umbrella in control.

So we can look at occupation from the point of view of energy and effort—how much energy certain activities use and how much re-charge energy they give back. This is the third dimension of our occupational umbrella—the handle. You need to learn how to hold the handle so the spokes and canopy point in the right direction, to control the umbrella against a gust of wind and to make adjustments before the umbrella blows inside out. You'll value having the right amount of energy when you want it and when you need it.

When looking at the energy of a task, it is important to conceptually understand the difference between physical energy and emotional energy. The physical energy is the effort needed to move, balance, coordinate, and think to do things. The emotional energy is the effort needed to decide what to do, to get started, to keep going, to face the challenges, and to risk not achieving the result you would like. Physical effort is easily measured—you can measure your heart rate, breathing rate and oxygen levels as an indication of muscle effort and fatigue. Physical effort can be modified by doing things differently—part of exploring the ingredients of tasks in the previous chapter. But we don't often think about emotional energy as something that is tangible, measurable, or controllable. In this chapter we'll explore some ideas about measuring and taking control of your emotional energy levels.

Energy load and energy re-charge

Different tasks and different ways of doing things take different amounts of energy to get started and to keep going until you finish. The physical effort of starting a petrol lawn mower, checking fuel levels, adjusting the choke, pumping the fuel, and pulling the start cord (numerous times!) is very different to the effort of plugging in an electric mower or getting the hand mower out of the shed. But the effort of keeping going with a hand mower is greater than for a powered mower, and a very different type of physical effort to what is needed to operate a ride-on mower.

The emotional energy needed to get started and to keep going is not always so obvious, and sometimes tricky to separate from the physical effort. Starting to mow the lawn the day after the mower has been serviced compared to when you've had nothing but trouble the last couple of times is likely to be very different.

Another example is to look at the simple task of getting up in the morning. We all know there are days when getting out of bed is sooo much harder, and yet each day it's the same physical activity. Knowing what the day ahead holds has a big influence: getting up when you are heading off to a music festival compared to having a dentist's appointment to have your wisdom teeth removed; children getting up on Christmas morning compared to a school day; waking with pain and stiffness instead of feeling refreshed. These are all varying emotional contexts that create very different emotional loads for getting started with the same task.

Activities also give back energy—the satisfaction of success, the inherent pleasure of hobbies, the relief of knowing "it's done". As you keep going with an activity, you use varying amounts of physical and emotional energy; but these energies are off-set by the re-charge of satisfaction and pleasure as you are doing the task. I play the clarinet, and there's a certain amount of effort needed to move my fingers and breathe and blow and hold my mouth in exactly the right position. But sitting in the middle of an orchestra playing a symphony is pure magic—I feel no effort at all. It gives me an enormous burst of energy and for several hours after a rehearsal (let alone a concert) I'm buzzing. Even the more mundane daily tasks can give back some energy as we do them. Having a bath or shower can itself be pleasurable as well as something that has to be done. Some people find mowing the lawn very satisfying to see the emerging results of keeping their yard in check. Baking can be energising for some people, for others it is calming, and for some people it is pure frustration and energy-sapping.

So what is it that determines the emotional energy levels of tasks for different people at different times and stages of life? If you look at the above examples of mowing the lawn and getting out of bed, you will see that it is the meaning, purpose, and expected outcome that generate the energy load and determine the emotional effort needed to get going and keep going.

In other words, it is your umbrella canopy that largely determines the emotional load, mixed with your confidence in what you are doing and how important it is for you at the time.

The amount of re-charge energy you get, both during the task and when it is finished, relates to your satisfaction and enjoyment—how well you think you are going while you are doing the task, how enjoyable the task itself is, and the satisfaction you derive from the final result. These are the results of the interactions between your umbrella spokes. The umbrella spokes largely determine the re-charge factor.

Graphing emotional energy

Our energy levels fluctuate throughout the day and the week as we do things and contemplate what we've done. It always takes at least some emotional energy to get started and varying amounts of energy to keep going as the energy load interacts with our pleasure and satisfaction re-charge.

You can picture your energy levels as a fluctuating, wavy line in-between two parallel horizontal lines. The horizontal lines represent the two extremes of emotional energy—too much is when thoughts and behaviour become chaotic, uncontrolled and unpredictable and too little is when life is bleak and doing anything at all is overwhelming and effortful. An example that we've all seen of the top line—of being over-aroused and highly emotional—is an overexcited child who has so much energy and excitement bursting out that they are unable to control what they are doing. When some people reach this level, they shut down completely and become "paralysed" by their fears and thoughts and emotions; others become very disorganised and erratic. This is the time you may act impulsively or irrationally and make decisions that you later regret.

The bottom line—representing lack of emotional energy—is the line that will be familiar to anyone who has had depression. It is the point at which it is too effortful to get started with anything, too hard to get out of bed in the morning, and the simplest task becomes overwhelming.

In between the two lines, the energy level dips when you start an activity from the effort needed to get started. At some point your energy level starts to increase as your pleasure and satisfaction kick in. For some activities this isn't until the task is finished; for others it's almost immediate as your pleasure re-charge overtakes the emotional load of keeping going.

When we are fit and well, our energy levels oscillate up and down but mostly stay well clear of the extremes. Daily life chugs along without consciously thinking about emotional energy. Over the course of a day, a week, a month our energy levels reach an equilibrium as we do things to recuperate, to re-energise, to calm and soothe.

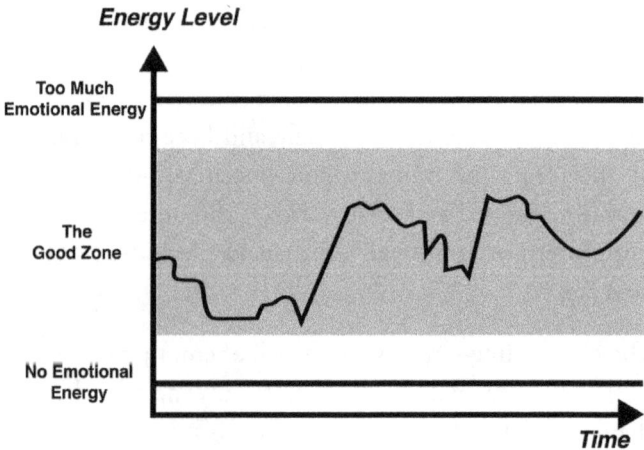

When the graph shifts

When life becomes challenging, when we are faced with long-term health issues, when our circumstances are not what we wanted or had hoped for, the whole graph shifts downwards or the waves increase in size to look (and feel) like a rollercoaster.

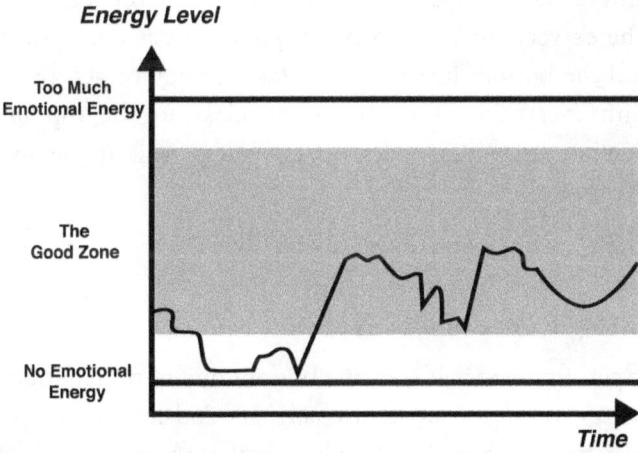

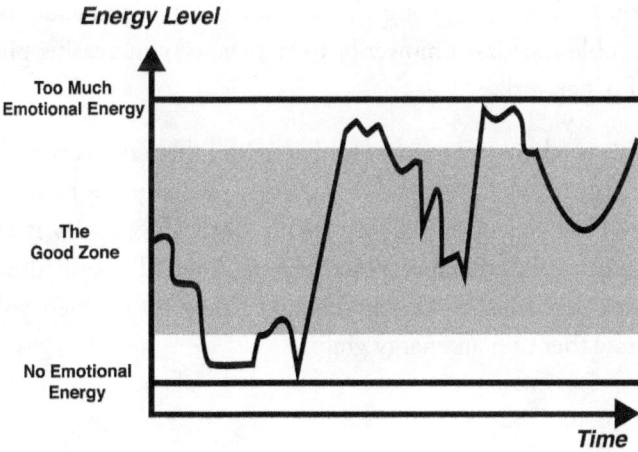

This means you are constantly closer to the extremes. There's very little gap between your current energy level and the bottom line and yet it takes energy to get started with everything. Or you are so close to the top line that any enjoyment and re-charge you get will tip you into overflow.

Taking a dose of energy

If you find yourself near the bottom line of no emotional energy, regardless of what challenges and limitations you face, getting started with doing anything becomes in itself a huge challenge. Anything that takes a large amount of energy to get started will deplete you of all energy and stop you from keeping going. This is not the time to tackle the troublesome lawn mower or to face the ever-increasing pile of paperwork.

This is when you need to find activities that take very little energy to get started and that quickly re-charge your energy levels as you do them. My friend Chris Coop, who is an occupational therapist practising in Townsville, calls these "tick activities" as this is the shape they form when you draw them on an energy graph.

Energy Level

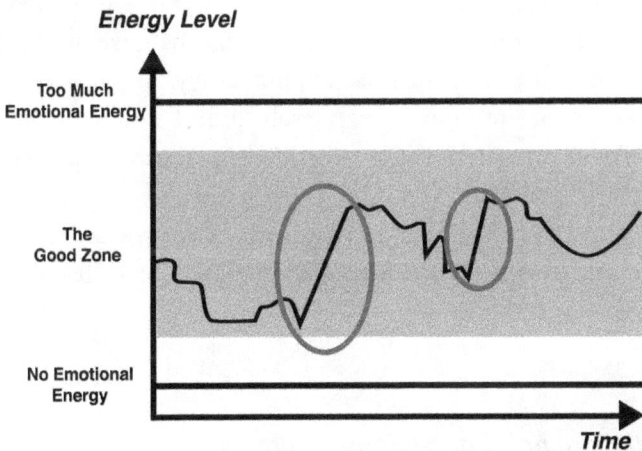

Tick activities are very individualised and sometimes not what you would expect. They are activities that take no preparation (or are already set up), they rely on no-one else but yourself (and therefore are by default something you do by yourself), and that start to give an overall energy boost within five to ten minutes.

There's an activity in Chapter 7 that helps you work through the process of graphing your energy levels for different activities to discover which activities are tick activities for you at this point in time. This activity will also help you become more aware of your emotional energy levels at different times of the day and to know when you might need to take a 'dose of energy' with a tick activity.

Once you discover your "tick activities", you can deliberately use them to recharge your energy graph (your batteries); to bring you back towards the centre of the graph so you have enough energy reserves to do the things that give meaning and pleasure but which also require energy. As you become more aware of your energy levels and of how particular tasks or activities change your levels, you can adapt what you do and when you do it to have more control of your energy through the day and the week. When you are feeling low on energy, you can take an energy dose with one of your tick activities.

Hook handles on your umbrella

All my illustrations of umbrellas have hook handles to remind you that it is meaning, purpose, and pleasure that hooks you into actually doing things. The handle and spokes connect directly to your umbrella canopy. You won't suddenly find everything you do fun and enjoyable; there will always be things that simply need to be done. But by more clearly understanding why you are doing them, and making changes so that you use the least amount of energy possible for your daily grind, you will have more energy for the fun parts of your day. As you learn to hold the handle in different ways i.e. take back control of your emotional energy levels, you will find yourself being hooked into doing more of the things that bring meaning, purpose and pleasure to your day.

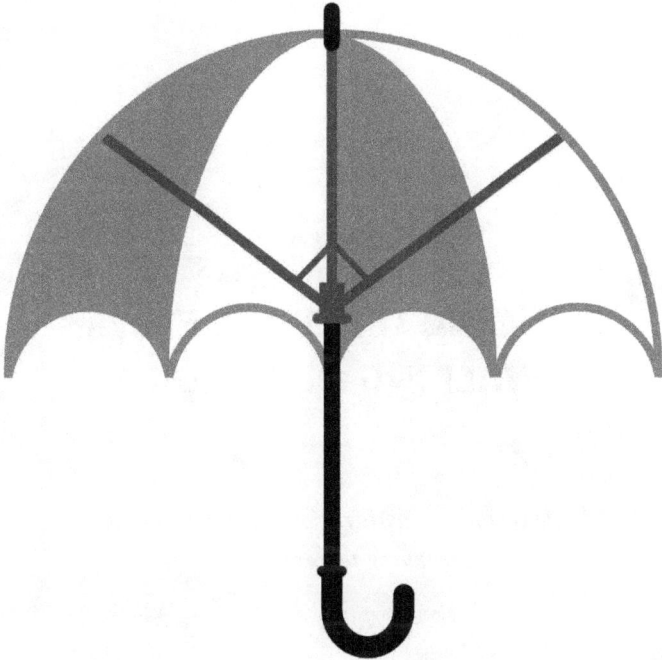

Chapter 5

BRINGING IT ALL TOGETHER—
WALKING IN THE RAIN

"Life isn't about waiting for the storm to pass, it's about learning to dance in the rain."

—*Vivian Greene*

Occupational engagement—the whole umbrella

This model of daily living **Bit by Bit** all comes together when the component parts of your umbrella (the things you do and their meaning, the ingredients and their interactions, and energy) are brought together to form a complete picture. This is what the literature calls occupational engagement—not simply doing things (participating), but engaging in the deeper meaning and wider context of daily living activities.

While it is important to understand which tasks need to be done each day to maintain your health and wellness (survival), this alone won't help you (re)engage in your everyday life. It is the meaning and purpose you ascribe to the things you do within the context of your current stage of life, combined with ensuring that you have all four domains covered, that will hook you into actually engaging in daily life. Matching the meaning of what you do to your aspirations and values, and engaging in activities that have purpose and inspire you, will generate vitality to create a life (style) that works for you.

This is why filling in a checklist of "Can you do . . . ?" in isolation from the context of your life won't help you move forward. The umbrella approach to daily living is so much more than simply "doing". It relates to feeling safe and secure; deliberately and consistently being able to do things that give meaning, purpose, and pleasure to your life; doing them easily, efficiently, consistently, in good time and in such a way that you derive enjoyment and satisfaction from the process itself as well as the outcome. This occupational engagement shapes your every day life to give you meaning, purpose, and pleasure.

Rain as life's challenges and experiences

Now that you have explored the make-up of your umbrella, let's extend the analogy to include the rain and streetscape.

We can start with looking at the rain as life's experiences and challenges. Have you ever been caught out in the rain, been drenched before you've had time to look for a dry shelter, or been out in the open with no shelter, umbrella, rain-coat, or anything to use as a make-shift cover? If you've had an unexpected illness or accident, or experienced a traumatic event or life crisis, this is often what the first few weeks or months feel like. Blindsided and taken by surprise, you scramble to gather information and help. There are other times in life when we are prepared for the rain—umbrella at the ready. Sometimes life's experiences and changes are planned or we have some warning—but that doesn't mean we have to like the fact that it is raining and it doesn't change the fact that we need to deal with the rain.

Changing streetscape over time

Imagine walking down the street (with or without an umbrella) as you are moving through the changing streetscape of your life. Conceptually, the streetscape changes as you walk through each individual task and also from a life-long perspective of the evolving nature of your roles and routines that occur at different ages and stages of life.

Your personal skills change over time. Throughout childhood, your skills change and reshape through each of the developmental stages; in adulthood, you face the challenges of and learn from your work experiences, your family life, and community connections. Personal skills and abilities continually change as your life and lifestyles evolve. Today you are the sum of your life's experiences; tomorrow you will be different.

The environments in which you operate change as well. You may live in several different homes and cities throughout your life. Your social circles change; people with whom you live change as families take shape and as children move away from home. Your economic circumstances undergo several evolutions at different stages of your life. Larger, societal types of influences, such as political and cultural contexts also unfold to shape your daily life.

The things that you do in everyday life also change at different ages and stages of life. Your routines, habits, and rituals change over the course of your life as do the roles you take on. Life as a singleton, as part of a couple, as a parent, an empty-nester, a worker, a retiree—these roles all demand different tasks and skills and connections with people. The daily life of a university student is very different to the everyday routines of a full-time worker. The ways in which you connect with people change over your lifespan as do your interests, hobbies, and leisure pursuits.

The streetscape of life is constantly evolving—sometimes predictably, sometimes unexpectedly and not always how we would like. Some people say that having a major injury or illness, particularly one that results in a life-long diagnosis, is like being lifted out of the world you know into a landscape that is foreign and uncertain. The old familiar ways of doing things no longer work. You haven't yet learnt to predict the day's weather. Will it rain or not? Will you be able to hold the umbrella against the swirling winds?

During a major life event or crisis, the immediacy of financial arrangements, appointments, fear of the unknown future, illness, hospitals, re-routing daily routines, all take over daily life in the short term. As the crisis abates, you are often left feeling that life is in some way deficient, unsatisfying, not as you had hoped it would become. Everyday seems as if you are walking out in the rain without an umbrella; not being able to find an umbrella that will provide at least some shelter and respite. You find yourself having to choose between getting soaking wet and not going out at all.

Responses to the rain—opportunities for change

In the film 'Notting Hill', there's a lovely scene of the market place throughout the changing seasons with people going about their daily tasks as the seasons progress, to denote time passing in the story line. It shows the same people wearing different clothes in the different seasons, their postures change as they stoop against the wind and scurry through the street in the winter rain where they were previously leisurely walking and talking during the summer days. Different postures, different movements, different clothes, different colours. Same tasks, same people, same market street.

When it rains, we go about our day differently. We change what we wear; we walk at a different speed; we take different things with us. But our essential being hasn't changed. Our values and our aspirations remain the same.

When exploring all the component parts to your umbrella, you will realise there is much greater scope for change than you previously thought. The first opportunity for change is in exploring what you actually do and how you spend your time. By understanding why you do things and clarifying the intent and the hoped-for outcome, you can ensure that you cover all four domains equally. You can also look for different things to do that achieve the same meaning and purpose. Look for any imbalance in your umbrella canopy as this will help you target what is most important at this particular time and how to prioritise what you do each day.

The second opportunity for change is to look at the ingredients of each task. You have more options for change when you look beyond your personal skills and capabilities and look at the environmental factors and the task characteristics. Each change you make needs to have a direct line—a spoke—to the intent of what you are doing, not just a means to complete the task.

And lastly, you can look at the energy components of the tasks—their individual energy load and re-charge, as well as the cumulative energy graph over time.

This fundamentally changes the way you go about change. From this perspective, you work downwards from the canopy of meaning to look at the ingredients (the spokes) that support the umbrella and what changes can be made to them to change the outcome. Starting with the canopy can help you focus on the reason and intention of your activities instead of the old familiar ways of doing things. You can build your confidence by trying different types of spokes—to swap some of the spokes that used to work for you for new spokes that now work better. And you can monitor your emotional energy levels needed to hold the umbrella securely.

Carrying this umbrella can lessen the impact of the challenges that life has imposed on you. It won't necessarily stop you from getting wet and doesn't always keep you entirely dry. But it will shield you from the worst of the rain. This should form the basis of every change you make to your daily life—any task, exercise, treatment or therapy that you do needs to relate directly back to one of the meaning and purpose domains—the words or colours on your umbrella canopy.

Looking at occupational engagement in this way ensures your umbrella is colourful, is large enough to provide sufficient cover for the amount of rain (if you are in a tropical downpour you'll definitely need a golf umbrella), the spokes are strong enough and plentiful enough to stop the umbrella blowing inside out in the wind, and the handle is shaped for you to have a firm grip and sufficient energy to hold it securely while pointing the umbrella into the wind to reduce the effort needed.

Your occupational umbrella can help you see things in a different light and discover new possibilities.

This is the start of your journey. Let's start to look at the colours and shape of your umbrella and create your own personalised umbrella assessment.

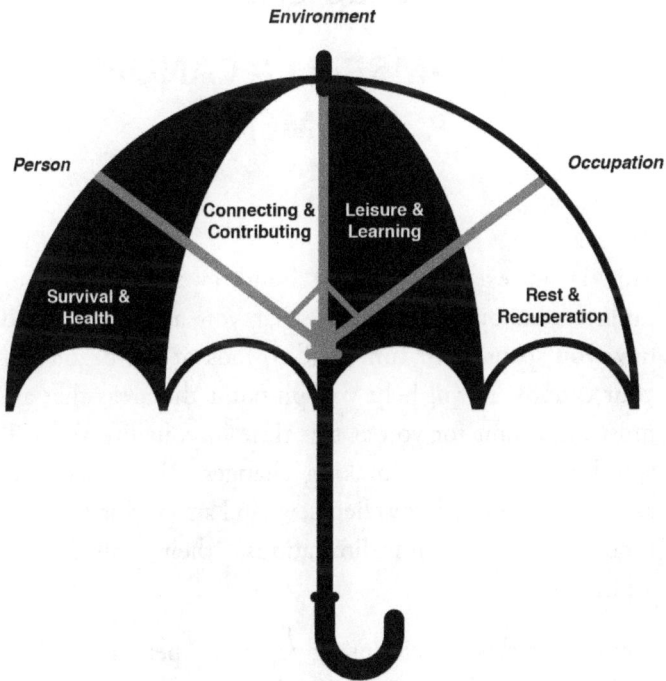

Chapter 6

YOUR UMBRELLA CANOPY ASSESSMENT

This is an exercise to help build awareness of your umbrella canopy, to explore what you actually do and how you spend your time, and to look at the balance of your canopy. It will help you pinpoint the areas that are most important for you at this time in your life and will simplify how to start making changes. This is the first assessment I do with my clients, when I am getting to know their challenges and limitations, their values and aspirations.

You can do this exercise using paper and pen, a bunch of sticky notes or electronically. Sticky notes on a table top or wall can make it easier to shift different tasks into different categories as you explore your occupations.

Coloured felt pens, highlighters or pencils will be useful but not essential. Likewise, you might choose to use different font styles and colours electronically to help sort your tasks.

Getting started

1. First, answer the general question: *What do you do on a typical day?*

Jot down some notes—a mini brain storm—in no particular order. Create an overall representation of a typical day, not a detailed list at this stage.

Points to consider:

- When answering this question, don't restrict yourself to thinking about today or yesterday. What is your impression of a run-of-the-mill day for you?

- What are the things that you generally do throughout the day?

- What marks it as a typical day?

- Even if you think you don't have any specific daily routines, there are some things that you do most days: get up, get dressed. Do you have a shower in the morning or the evening? Do you usually have a main meal in the middle of the day or the evening?

- What do you do to fill your day?

Write down all the things that come to mind.

Some people are tempted to create a timeline of daily routines. This can be a useful cue to think more broadly about roles and habits, but may not represent the full picture of daily routines, particularly if you are recovering from an illness or injury or are "out of routine". Perhaps begin with a general sense or picture of your days and think about them from an ***occupation*** point of view rather than time-based.

This will not be an exhaustive list of everything you have ever done in your life. Nor will it be a complete list of your current routines and habits. It is simply a starting point, to begin investigating the meaning and purpose of the things you do that occupy your time. The things that are uppermost in your mind at this point in time.

2. ***Next jot down the less frequent things you do:***
   - Where do you go throughout the week, and what do you do there?
   - What groups, clubs, activities, sports, meetings, and social events do you attend weekly or monthly?
   - What do you do on the spur of the moment?
   - What are your "doing nothing" times?

3. *Now think about what is the highlight of your day, of your week, and the month for you.*

- What are you doing when you feel happiest and at your best?

- What do you do for pleasure?

- What are your hobbies, interests, amusements and recreation?

- What do you do when you are on holidays, away from your usual daily grind?

Try not to think too much about it. Write down your first response to these questions. In psychological circles, we generally say the first response is the right one. What that means is that your first gut response is what you are thinking about at the moment; what's high on your radar and high on your list of what is important to you at this point in time.

4. *Then jot down the low point of the week*

Again, don't over-think it; write down your first response.

If you were to do this exercise in a couple of days or next week, it's highly likely you would have a very different first response. But that doesn't matter because your umbrella will evolve over time; you can redo this exercise at any time. Don't get stuck on pondering about whether what you've actually written down is the most important; it's simply what is uppermost in your mind at this moment—what you worry about, are concerned about, are frustrated about or what pleases you and gives you the most satisfaction and enjoyment at this point in time. These are the things that are uppermost in your mind and they are often the best place to start in terms of changing the things you do that occupy your time.

5. *You may like to list some of the things you have previously done that have occupied your time*

- What are the things you really miss doing?

- What gave you a strong sense of fulfilment and purpose or intense enjoyment that you no longer do?

- What are you glad to not be doing any more?

Note which are past activities—use a particular colour or a different font or use a different coloured sticky note to highlight previous activities.

You should now have a good list of things you do in your daily life.

Sorting your umbrella canopy

Up to this point, all you've done is simply made a list of things you do that fill your day. It's time to sort your list into the four umbrella categories of survival and health, connecting and contributing, leisure and learning, and rest and recuperation.

If you are using pen and paper, grab a new sheet of paper and divide it into 4 sections. If you are using sticky notes, clear a section of table and write a sticky note heading for each category. If you are doing this exercise electronically, create a new document or section with four columns.

6. ***Go through your list and look at each task individually. Decide whether or not the task or activity is a survival and health task.***

- Is this something you need to do in order to maintain your health and stay alive?

- What would happen if you didn't do it? (Would you eventually become ill?)

Move all your survival and health tasks into a distinct column or section. Move the sticky notes to one section of the table; or write these tasks in a column headed survival and health; or electronically cut and paste them into a section of your document. This will create a distinct area of your umbrella canopy.

Points to consider:

- Remember that tasks and activities can sometimes be in more than one category. If a particular task has a meaning or purpose beyond your own health (e.g. cooking, as previously described) put it in the survival and health category, and mark it as potentially belonging in another category as well.

- If you're not sure if something belongs in survival, the chances are it belongs there as well as in one of the other categories.

7. Sort the rest of your list into the remaining three categories.

Look at each task or activity individually. Think very carefully about why you do a particular task, the intention behind the task for you within the context of your life. What is the reason for passing time in this way? Remember that the categories represent the meaning and purpose of what you do, not how well you achieve the desired result.

- Is it something through which you **contribute** to the world around you, to your household, to the community, to the wellbeing of family or friends?

- Is it something that **connects** you to other people?

- Do you **learn** new things? Do you as a person expand as a result of doing this activity each time or over time?

- Is there an inherent pleasure or **leisure** from simply doing this activity?

- Does this task or activity help you **recuperate** from the melee of daily life?

- Does it soothe you, enable you to get outside of your thoughts and worries, to ***rest*** and be in a headspace of calm?

- Do you feel energised and revitalised after doing this activity (***recuperation***)?

- Re-write all the tasks that belong in more than one category. Include them in each of the relevant categories.

Points to consider:

Keep in mind that if you do something with other people, it doesn't necessarily fall into the category of connecting and contributing. There are some things that you need to do to stay healthy that you tend to do with other people without it necessarily providing a meaningful connection. For example, going shopping /to the supermarket and engaging in the social pleasantries with the shop assistant may not necessarily serve as a way of connecting you with your community. It may simply be acknowledging the social mores of society. Or it may be a very important part of connecting with the people around you, and which afterwards gives you a very strong sense of having done something more than simply buying milk and bread.

When categorising your family daily routines, be mindful of which tasks affect your own health and wellbeing (survival and health) and which ones form part of your role as parent and, therefore, contribute to your children's health and wellbeing (the contributing and connecting category). Some tasks, such as preparing a family meal fall into both categories.

There are no right or wrong categories. Your umbrella canopy is your perspective, your context, your intention. Don't overthink the categories; go with your gut response as to which broad meaning or purpose fits the task.

Balancing your umbrella canopy

8. *Place all 4 categories next to each other, so you can see them all at the same time*

Take a broad overview of the umbrella canopy. When looking at your four sections, what is your gut response to the following questions?

- Is where you spend the most time and energy the most important?

- Do you have a balance of things that you must do and that you do for pleasure?

- Do you do things that re-energise you to counter the things that are fatiguing?

- Is there a good balance between all 4 domains or is it heavily weighted to 1 or 2 of the categories?

- Which category needs more and/or which could do with less?

9. *Choose a category to analyse.*

Look at that particular domain as a whole (as a group of things you do).

- How well do you manage these tasks overall?

- Do they take too much time and energy with respect to the things you would prefer to do?

- Do they achieve the meaning and purpose you intend?

- Do you feel safe, confident, and satisfied when you do these activities?

- Are they easy to do?

- Do you feel comfortable? Do they cause pain?

- Do you actually do these things consistently when you need or want to?

- How has your illness, injury or reason for seeking out this book affected your ability to do these tasks?

- What has changed? Is the change sudden, or has it happened gradually?

- What are the most important? The most satisfying? The most fun?

Make a few general notes. You don't need to specifically answer each question—make notes about the questions that are most relevant or that resonate with you at this point in time. Remember that tomorrow, next week, and next month you can go through this same exercise with a different focus or with renewed understanding of the different domains as they relate to your specific lifestyle. And likely come up with different results. So concentrate on what is uppermost in your mind today.

10. If you were to make one change in this category, what/where would it be?

Return to the meaning and purpose of this category. What one thing would you like to do differently, more easily, safely, to achieve the reason and intention of the activity?

Always remember, when thinking about making changes, don't start with a task. Start with the meaning and purpose.

Opening your umbrella

This exercise helps clarify the overarching meaning and purpose of the things you do within your context at this point in time. It can help you recognise where there is an imbalance in your umbrella canopy, and it creates a reference point for any changes or exercises or activities that you do.

Rebalancing your umbrella can be the first step towards reclaiming meaning, purpose and pleasure in everyday life. It can help you start to thrive rather than simply survive. As you become more attuned to the intent of what you do each day, particularly in terms of the four domains, you can focus on creating balance throughout each day and over the course of a week and a month. This will also help you separate the concepts of meaning and purpose (the canopy) from satisfaction and pleasure with the outcome (the spokes).

The umbrella canopy exercise is the start of an occupational therapy journey, that guides you through exploring and changing your canopy, spokes and handle, bit by bit. The canopy exercise is the initial assessment; exploring how and where to make changes is the next step. The Emotional Energy Dose Activity in the next chapter is one way you make changes to the handle of your umbrella. If you would like to further analyse and change the canopy, spokes and handle of your umbrella, go to the workable living website at www.workableliving.com.au to see the latest resources available.

To finish your umbrella assessment, draw an umbrella canopy around your word lists.

Chapter 7

EMOTIONAL ENERGY DOSE ACTIVITY

The Emotional Energy Dose Activity is a structured exercise designed to boost your emotional energy levels. You will learn how to measure your emotional energy levels, and how to measure energy changes after doing specific activities. This will help you discover which activities will consistently give you a boost—a dose of energy. It is an exercise that will take you about half an hour to set up, and then takes 10 minutes once or twice a day for two or three weeks while you discover your personalised energy dose. You can then choose to take a five or ten minute energy dose each day, or as needed throughout the week.

Someone who has diabetes checks their blood sugar levels regularly throughout the day, to determine whether they need more insulin, and what foods they need to eat to keep their blood sugars at a healthy level. Managing blood sugar levels is a very individualised process—it takes time working with a health team to work out how someone's body will respond to different foods and different doses of insulin, especially when first diagnosed. Over time this can change; it needs to be reviewed at regular intervals.

Similarly, when energy levels are in short supply, you can check your emotional levels throughout the day, and use specific 'doses' of activity to help restore equilibrium. As with diabetes, this needs some initial investigation, it will take some tweaking to find what works well for you, and will need to be reviewed as your life continues to evolve.

Use the Emotional Energy Worksheet at the end of this chapter, or download a copy at http://workableliving.com. au/download/EEworksheet.pdf Print a copy, or have it easily accessible as an editable electronic document.

Getting started

1. *Choose the right 'word' to measure*

The first step is to decide exactly what it is that you are going to measure, or more precisely, what words will prompt you to easily tap into your energy levels.

For some people, simply asking "What is your emotional energy on a scale of 1 to 10?" is the only cue they need. For others, this is too nebulous and they need words that are more personalised to their own situation. Think about the

words and language you use to describe your daily life—
what are terms that you tend to use that are meaningful
for you?

- How do you feel when you've just finished
  doing the highlight of your week or month?

- What do you do for pleasure? Describe how you
  feel when doing this activity.

- Go back to your umbrella canopy exercise—
  pick the most fun or satisfying activity in each
  category, and think about how you feel when
  doing it or when it's finished.

Choose words that describe how you feel when you are at
your best. Happy, enthusiastic, full of energy, real good,
in a good mood, contented, on top of the world are some
phrases that people have used. Find a word that resonates
with you, at this point of time.

2. *Next, choose the opposite word*

Think about what the opposite would be. If 'full of energy'
or 'feeling real good' is a 10/10, what words describe 1/10?

Pretty low, down, lacklustre, not good and weary are some
words that might describe how you feel.

When choosing your words, make sure they relate to
energy, vitality or mood at this stage of your life and not
your overall life satisfaction. During this exercise you need

to concentrate on your emotional energy reserves, not life satisfaction.

3.   *Write the words you have chosen over the 1 and 10 of the measuring scale at the top of the chart*

Emotional Energy Worksheet

(your words)------------------------FEELING------------------------(your words)

1	2	3	4	5	6	7	8	9	10

4.   *Choose a time of day and set a reminder*

Next, decide on a time of day when you are most likely to be able to set aside five or ten minutes of uninterrupted time.

This is often trial and error. You might like to start with two different times of the day. When you chart the exercise over the first couple of weeks, you will quickly see which times work best for you and which time slots remain empty.

Initially it is best to have a consistent time(s) of the day, so that when you measure energy levels before and after an activity you know that it is the activity itself that produces any change and isn't being affected by the time of day.

Set a reminder to do the exercise, something that will jog your memory at the particular time of day you have chosen—a sticky note on your wardrobe door, a fridge note or a reminder app on your phone.

5. *Now choose activities to put on your list*

These are activities that you find enjoyable, but there are three very important characteristics of the activities for this exercise:

a. It involves no-one else at any stage. This is exclusively about you and your energy levels at a particular point in time. The activity can't rely on someone else being available, nor on it being influenced by someone else who is willing, able, or enjoying themselves at that particular time. It needs to be entirely you by yourself.

b. It is something that will only take 10 minutes to complete or that you can stop after 10 minutes and still feel a level of satisfaction or achievement.

c. It is something that is readily available at the time and place you choose for this exercise. It requires little energy and effort to start. Initially you may need to organise your activities so they are ready for use—new art or craft supplies, buying a jigsaw and mat to fold it away, stocking up on library books, dusting off the running shoes . . .

In other words, these will be "tick activities" that also fit the above three criteria.

Hints for finding appropriate activities

- Look at what you put in the leisure and learning category of your umbrella assessment; also the rest and recuperation domain.

- What is the highlight of your day, week, and month?

- What did you note as being important, creative, re-energising? Can you adapt these activities to match the above criteria?

- Are there aspects of connecting with other people that you can prepare ahead by yourself? For example, a lady who lived in a rural area liked to have a stock of gifts for her grandchildren's birthdays. One of the tasks on her list was to spend 10 minutes on the internet looking for gift ideas, particularly mail-order items. Another person spent 10 minutes looking through recipe books in preparation for family dinners.

- These should be activities that you don't have to do, or that may need to be done in the future but at this point in time you are doing for pleasure.

- Be specific about the activity. For example, if you choose reading as an activity, "10 minutes reading" is very vague. Specify what you will read—fiction, newspaper, poetry, a particular blog. And perhaps prescribe where you will read—in the garden, on the balcony, in your favourite arm chair.

- Be careful about the subject matter you read, watch or listen to. Dark themes and intensely emotive topics are unlikely to lift your spirits.

- Be very specific about whether the activity is timed, or based on how much you do, e.g. read for 10 minutes vs. read one chapter. This is important for the later stages of the exercise—knowing exactly how much time it will take and exactly what you need to do to change/improve your energy levels.

- The tasks can be active or sedentary, indoor or outdoor. Having a mix is good (but not essential) so you have options for different moods at your chosen time of day.

Develop a first list of six or eight activities. Any more, and you may initially have difficulty choosing between them. Having too few on your list may leave you not being in the mood for any of them on a particular day.

Each of the activities must fit all three of the above criteria.

Remember that this initial list is a trial list that you will use to collect data about your emotional energy levels. It is a list that you will continue to change as you recognise what works for you at any particular stage of your life.

6. Set up your activities and measuring chart so they are easily accessible and ready for use.

Write your initial list of activities on the chart; make sure your chart is easily accessible.

Gather any supplies, equipment or resources you need for each of the activities. Think about having an Emotional Energy tool box or folder or basket for your supplies, activities list and energy chart. Pick a specific place to store your resources or a specific folder or desk-top icon if your activities and chart are electronic.

Collecting data

During the first couple of weeks you will be collecting data to find out what works and what doesn't work for you— what you don't do is equally as informative as what you actually get around to doing. Don't worry about whether you think it is working or not—you are simply collecting data.

7. At your designated time, choose one activity from your list

When your timer goes off or at the designated time, fetch your measuring chart and choose an activity from your list.

Don't spend time choosing. Just pick one activity; and if necessary take the one at the top of the list.

Write the activity in the first column and note the time of day on the chart.

8. *Measure your emotional level on a scale of 1 to 10 at this point in time*

On a scale of 1 to 10, with the words you have chosen to denote the extremities, how do you feel right now? Note this number on your chart next to the start time.

Don't over think it—just write down your initial response.

For this exercise, it doesn't matter where you start on the scale. The aim of the exercise is to find activities that show a change of emotional energy after 10 minutes; activities that raise you one or two notches on your scale. The starting point is immaterial.

Also note that 10/10 is not where you would expect to be every day—this is for the major events of the year, special celebrations and significant milestones.

9. *Spend 10 minutes doing the activity*

Be pedantic about timing the activity or doing the specified amount of your activity. Then stop to take your next emotional energy measurement.

10. *Immediately after the activity, measure your emotional energy level again.*

On a scale of 1 to 10, how do you feel now? Write the number and the current time in the final two columns.

Don't analyse the result. Don't fret about whether it "works" or not; simply record your data.

If you want to keep going with your activity after your 10 minutes, that's fine. But make sure you record your energy level at the 10 minute mark.

11. Rinse and repeat

Repeat this process of collecting data once or twice a day.

I recommend charting activities for seven to ten days before looking over the information you have collected. If it's really obvious that some of the activities don't fit the criteria for this exercise, then explore different options by revisiting the activity choices above. And likewise, play with the time of day if you find your initial choice just isn't working. But mostly you should just collect the data; acknowledging that what doesn't work or doesn't get done is useful information for the next stage of analysing your data.

Analysing your data

12. Finding a consistent time

Look at the column where you have recorded the time of day.

- Which time appears most frequently? Is there a stand out time of day when you were most frequently able to do the exercise?

- Is one of your trial times of day noticeably absent?

If you have tried two or three different times of the day, the chart will likely show which time is the most consistent or convenient. Any times that are charted on three or less days of the week are unlikely to work as a consistent time for a daily dose of energy.

Ideally you will find a time of day when you have charted an activity session on five or more days of the week. If not, think about other times of your daily routine now that you are more familiar with how the exercise works. Try to find a consistent time as 'daily doses' are best taken at the same time each day.

If, over a few weeks, you try several different times throughout the day and none seems to be consistent, you may need to think about a rolling schedule throughout the week. If all else fails, set your time as either immediately you get up or last thing before going to bed, regardless of the actual time.

13. Creating an energy dose activity list

Look at your emotional energy numbers pre-activity and post-activity. Highlight the rows where there is an increase of 1 or 2 points.

- Is there an activity that consistently gives you a boost?

The aim is to find specific activities (specific "doses") that consistently lift you one or two notches higher on your chart, on the scale of 1 to 10. Remember it doesn't matter at what point on the scale you start the activity. You simply aim to improve one notch at a time.

You may need to do the data collection phase several times before you find a consistent result and a feasible list. The activities that give a good result—an increase of one or two notches—are often surprising and not what you would expect. So think laterally about choosing activities that fit the above three criteria.

If your results for a particular activity are very inconsistent but you'd like the activity to be on your list, try to be more specific about what you do. What was different about the activity when you had a good result in raising your emotional level? Re-read the sections in the ingredients chapter about the environment and task characteristics with this particular activity in mind, and think about which factors you can change for your next round of data collection.

This is a list that will develop over time. For some people, the same 10 or 12 items will work very effectively for the rest of their lives. For other people, the list will need to evolve as their life evolves. There will be tasks and activities that initially work but over time lose their ability to provide the benefit. And the time of day may also need to change. This isn't surprising considering what we have already discussed about daily habits and routines that change as our lifestyles and life stages evolve.

But for now, for the first month, develop your list of what works for you now. You can go through the process of developing a new list at any stage as you feel a need to change, add to, or mix up the tasks and activities.

Taking your daily dose of energy

Now that you have a time of day and list of activities, you don't need to chart your energy levels each day. Simply set your reminder and give yourself your daily dose of emotional energy activity at that time of day.

It's a good idea to take a few seconds to think about your current energy level on the 10-point scale to maintain the habit of conscious awareness of your emotions. As you become familiar with the practice of measuring your emotional levels on a regular basis, you will become more adept at recognising when you are approaching the bottom line of your overall energy graph. This is when you can choose one of your activity "doses" to remain above the line in addition to using this exercise on a regular (daily) basis to boost your energy charge.

Taking your daily dose will also remind you that you can now take control of your emotional energy. There is something you can **do** that is very concrete, very specific, is readily available, is entirely within your control, will only take 5 or 10 minutes, and will get you those extra one or two notches of satisfaction and energy.

However, don't think that if you do the task 10 times you'll be able to increase your energy level past 10. Nor will you be able to reach 10 by doing several activities one after the other/back to back. It won't work—and isn't the point of the exercise. This exercise is about boosting your emotional energy on a daily basis to help even out the roller-coaster curves of your cumulative energy graph. And for you to know that you can give yourself a "dose" of activity to move you one or two notches up the energy scale at any time, irrespective of your current energy level, the people around you, the environment you are in, or your current limitations.

You can repeat this process of analysing different activities to see which ones work for you at any time in the future. You can find new activities if the ones you've been using stop working for you, or if you would like more variety.

You will undoubtedly think of tick activities that recharge your energy but don't fit the three criteria for being a boost dose—in particular, tick activities that involve other people. While these activities don't fit this exercise of daily doses, they do fit the overarching umbrella model. Make sure you incorporate these into your weekly and monthly routines as these are the types of activities that ensure you have a good balance between the four domains of your umbrella while also re-energising you.

14. Finalising your energy dose kit

You are now ready to start taking your daily dose of emotional energy. Re-organise your kit of activities—re-stock your supplies, re-write your list, gather your resources and set your reminder. Your emotional energy kit is ready to use.

Emotional Energy Worksheet

(your words)----------------------FEELING----------------------(your words)

1	2	3	4	5	6	7	8	9	10

List of activities to choose from:

They must have the following characteristics:

- involve no-one else at any stage of the activity.
- can be done in 10 minutes or less, or can be stopped at the 10 minute mark.
- require very little energy and organisation to start.

Emotional Energy Worksheet

Activity	start time	energy level	end time	energy level

Chapter 8

MEANING, PURPOSE AND PLEASURE—BIT BY BIT

"Little by little, a little becomes a lot."

—*Tanzanian proverb*

The umbrella journey

We started this book taking a new look at normal everyday life, recognising that life doesn't always follow the path you'd like. The gradual meanderings of everyday living don't always lead to what you had expected or hoped; sometimes there are sudden twists and turns that steer you in unwanted directions. And all too often you are left thinking about what you could've, would've, should've done instead.

The umbrella model helps you see your daily life in a different light. The umbrella canopy, spokes and handle provide a new perspective. So let's retrace your steps through these theories and ideas and possibilities.

The umbrella canopy hones in on the meaning and purpose of what you do rather than the task or activity itself. How meaningful, worthwhile and enjoyable are the things you actually do during the day? And what of the things you don't do? We explored the interactions of all the factors that determine the outcome—the umbrella spokes. Not just your personal skills and capabilities, but the environments and task characteristics that provide new opportunities for change. Do you feel safe, comfortable, satisfied and inspired by what you achieve each day? And we then looked at energy levels (holding the umbrella handle) and how to monitor and manage the cumulative effects of energy. Do you have the right amount of energy when you want it and when you need it?

Changing the canopy

There are opportunities for change in each component of your umbrella. But with this model you can't start making changes until you've done some sort of umbrella canopy assessment. This is the crux of this approach. Start with your canopy of meaning and purpose, and as you work through the different domains and then downwards to the spokes and handle that hold up the canopy, what you do and how you do it will follow. As you start working with the umbrella model, you'll find that what you can and can't do becomes less significant than what you value and want to achieve in daily life. So many more possibilities will open up for you.

How did you go with your umbrella canopy assessment? What did it tell you?

Having a clearer picture of why you do things, and determining if the things you actually do each day have meaning and purpose for you at this stage of your life will lay the ground work for working with your canopy. It can be challenging to sort through an accumulation of habits and roles and activities, particularly if the reasons for doing them are lost in the mists of time. Sometimes the chaos of changed circumstances and an uncertain future can muddy your thoughts about what is important, valuable and inspiring for you. You may need more personalised help to complete the umbrella assessment, to clarify your values and re-discover the essence of who you are and what you want from life at this point in time. For some people, changed circumstances makes this all crystal clear, but that doesn't necessarily make it easy to move forward. Make your changes one at a time. If you rush ahead and make lots of changes all at once you won't know which of the changes worked for you. Also, change in itself takes energy—so be kind to yourself and take it little by little, bit by bit, to maintain control of your cumulative energy reserves.

Noting any gaps in your categories will help you direct your efforts to re-balancing your canopy, to make sure you are not spending all your time and energy on survival and health. You may discover that the ways you achieve meaning and purpose have changed or that the old ways no longer work. You might realise that you have different values and priorities than previously. These realisations will all help you prioritise where to spend your time and energy.

Take the first opportunity for change by balancing your umbrella canopy. Choose one category or occupation to work on at a time.

Adjusting the spokes

The next opportunity for change is with the spokes. The interactions of all the different spokes produce the outcome and give you pleasure, satisfaction and vitality (or not). Change one or two spokes and you can change the outcome to better match your intended meaning, purpose and pleasure. Once you decide on a specific part of your canopy to work on, you can start analysing the spokes of that particular occupation and how they relate to it's meaning and purpose.

There's a gargantuan amount of information that contributes to analysing your spokes. This includes all the main-stream health techniques and therapies that work on physical recovery and psychological health (person spokes), as well as delving into the plethora of environmental influences and task characteristics. This is the essence of occupational therapy—analysing the influences of the different ingredients and untangling all the interactions. For the moment it's important you take one small factor at a time, and make sure that any change you make has a direct link to the meaning and purpose of your umbrella canopy.

You can do a quick scan of your spokes to help pinpoint some strategies for change. Read the sections below that outline the spokes. Re-read the chapter on the ingredients of occupation with your particular task or purpose in mind. How can you apply the concepts to this particular occupation? How can you re-frame the examples so they relate to your circumstances? Which type of spoke— person, environment or occupation—will you target as the first point of change? Remember to change only one aspect at a time, one spoke at a time, so you can accurately gauge how effective and efficient the change has been. You only need to change one spoke to get a different outcome.

Person spokes

If you have had a recent accident, illness or a life-long diagnosis, you will probably already have spent a lot of time and effort working on your person spokes—on developing physical and cognitive skills and strategies. If this is the case, I strongly recommend you look at the other spokes as your first point of change, to take the pressure off your body and brain for now.

However, if you'd like to work on your person, I suggest starting with movement and body mechanics, especially if pain and energy are issues. The simplicity of using good body mechanics in all situations, not just when doing heavy lifting or challenging physical movements, can greatly improve pain and energy levels. Changing your postures and movement patterns throughout your whole day, and using the least amount of energy possible while protecting your body structures, will increase your safety and comfort while leaving more energy for the more pleasurable parts of your day.

Environment spokes

When looking at the environmental influences on a task or activity, think about the broad range of environments at play, not just the obvious ones. Think about the overall perspective of the physical ('built') environment in the community or in your home, as well as the small detail of how you set up a specific task. If reaching, bending, standing or stepping are difficult for you, changing the physical environment will likely help. Think also of sound and light and temperature; touch, taste and texture. Indoors or outdoors, with other people or by yourself. Are there parts of the sensory environment you can take away (the uncomfortable senses) or can you add soothing, comforting or energising sensations? What are the family, social and cultural influences that you might not have consciously thought about previously? Will a change in your emotional environment change the outcome? Will going to a different place or being with different people make a difference? Sometimes taking away some of the environmental factors can have a big impact without having to actively "change" something.

Occupation spokes

Working with occupational spokes is about teasing out the different ways of doing tasks and achieving your purpose. Watch how other people do things; ask your friends and family how they go about specific activities; challenge yourself to try a different way, now that you can consciously focus on meaning, purpose and pleasure instead of the task per se.

Is timing an important factor, and if so, how does this relate to the activity itself and the day as a whole? What single change can you make for it to be safer, more comfortable and easier on your body and brain? How important is it for you today, and therefore how much of your time and energy will you give this activity today?

You might look for different activities to achieve your purpose. And this circles straight back to the canopy: you need to be very clear of its meaning and purpose before you can choose a different activity that will achieve the result you want (and not simply replace a task with something that merely occupies your time).

What is your gut response to thinking about the type of ingredient that will be easiest to change? Think beyond the usual. If you are having difficulty pinpointing a particular spoke or ingredient, randomly choose a couple of factors from the examples in the ingredients chapter and challenge yourself to apply them to your chosen occupation.

Keep in mind that detailed strategies for working with spokes are not covered in this book—that's the subject of future books and resources. You can let me know which spokes you'd like to learn about at the Workable Living website www.workableliving.com.au

Holding firm to the handle

The third opportunity for change is with your umbrella handle, and the Emotional Energy Dose Activity is a great way to start. This takes a few weeks to systematically collect data on your own energy levels in order to create a daily dose of energy, so be patient with the exercise and yourself. Working with the handle component of your umbrella helps you measure, monitor and sustain your energy levels, so you have the right amount of energy when you want it and when you need it. The canopy creates the energy load; the interactions of the spokes provide the re-charge; and how you hold the handle monitors your cumulative energy use.

Balancing your umbrella canopy can help you re-think how you use your time and energy throughout the day and the week; and changing your spokes to find more efficient ways of doing things can help re-distribute your energy. Think of ways to use the least effort possible for your daily grind to save energy reserves for the more enjoyable aspects of your day. And include re-charge activities—the tick activities— regularly.

Unfurling your umbrella

You are now ready to unfurl your umbrella. In choosing to use an umbrella in everyday life, you can ensure you have good coverage across the entire canopy. You will have all four domains represented in your every day. Instead of spending all your time and energy on just surviving day to day, you will find ways of connecting with people around you and with your community, of having time and resources for leisure and learning, and opportunities to recuperate and re-energise.

You can be certain that your spokes will hold the canopy open. When you look down on an umbrella from above, you don't see the spokes. You don't know what they are made of or how many there are; but you know they are there holding the canopy open. Once you look beyond your person spokes to include the environments, different ways of doing things and different tasks, you open up a whole new range of ways to develop spokes that are numerous enough and strong enough to unfurl your umbrella. You can be confident in the strength of the scaffold they create. Ultimately it is the interaction of the spokes, working together to hold up the canopy, that provides pleasure and satisfaction.

You'll learn ways to firmly hold the hook handle of your umbrella. Understanding emotional energy, learning how to measure it and being more aware of it, discovering your tick activities and your calming activities, taking doses of energy (or calm) will better manage energy levels throughout the day and week.

You've started your umbrella journey. We've skimmed the surface of the umbrella approach in this book and I've given you a couple of tools to get started. There are lots more tools to customise your umbrella canopy in ways that suit your personal style and aspirations. There's a multitude of ways to change the spokes to keep it open. And innumerable tips on how to hold your umbrella against the prevailing weather conditions.

Think it through; delve into each of the umbrella components. Take it one step at a time. Get a handle on these concepts and you can look forward to making real change *Bit by Bit*.

ABOUT THE AUTHOR

I've been an occupational therapist for 30 years now, and have been privileged to work with people of all ages and stages of life. I have worked in hospitals, rehabilitation facilities and community settings; in home, office and industrial environments; in cities, country towns and remote communities.

I love that occupational therapy concentrates on the "doing" side of living. Life's experiences and everyday challenges change over time—often gradually and predictably; sometimes dramatically with no warning. My aim in writing this book is to lessen the impact these challenges impose on you, to find ways to enrich the valued aspects of your lifestyle.

I have reached the stage in my life when my children have left home, so I now have the freedom to move around and experience lifestyles in varied places. I like that this provides a benefit to my readers and clients—of providing flexibility for conversations and consultations. Just as I am not tied to a specific city and time zone, our connections are no longer tied to a clinic location and local business hours. I'd love to hear your thoughts about ***Bit by Bit***.

@workableliving

search for easy_daily_living

colleen@workableliving.com.au